THE LITTLE BOOK
OF HEALTH

Glenda Baum is a Chartered Physiotherapist who has held many positions in the Chartered Society of Physiotherapy. She has an MSc in Sports Physiotherapy and has sat on various national bodies advising on sport and exercise. Glenda is a health writer, best known for inventing Aquarobics on which she has written three acclaimed books, and gives lectures around the world on Aquatic Fitness. Glenda and her husband live in south-west London.

THE
LITTLE BOOK
OF
HEALTHY
FLYING

GLENDA BAUM

With illustrations by Jane Ancona

ARROW

Published by Arrow Books in 2001

1 3 5 7 9 10 8 6 4 2

Copyright © Glenda Baum 2001

Glenda Baum has asserted her right under the Copyright, Designs and
Patents Act, 1988 to be identified as the author of this work

First published in the United Kingdom in 2001 by Arrow Books

Arrow Books
The Random House Group Limited
20 Vauxhall Bridge Road, London, SW1V 2SA

Random House Australia (Pty) Limited
20 Alfred Street, Milsons Point, Sydney, New South Wales 2061, Australia

Random House New Zealand Limited
18 Poland Road, Glenfield, Auckland 10, New Zealand

Random House (Pty) Limited
Endulini, 5a Jubilee Road, Parktown 2193, South Africa

The Random House Group Limited Reg. No. 954009
www.randomhouse.co.uk

A CIP catalogue record for this book is available from the British Library

Papers used by Random House are natural, recyclable products made from
wood grown in sustainable forests. The manufacturing processes conform
to the environmental regulations of the country of origin

ISBN 0 09 943515 2

Design and make up by Roger Walker

Printed and bound in Denmark by
Nørhaven A/S, Viborg

To my high-flying husband, Harold,
our gorgeous grandchildren,
Leora, Micah, Ben, Joe and David,
and their wonderful parents

Introduction

Forty years ago, only the very wealthy could afford to fly regularly. Nowadays, for a variety of reasons, everybody seems to be doing it. Perhaps it's to visit family members who live in far-off countries; or maybe it's to attend a business meeting in a different country or even a different continent; or it could simply be for tourism. Whatever the reason, previously inaccessible parts of the world have been opened up to us all, and flying is both cheaper and faster than other means of travel for getting to distant parts of the world.

It is very much more comfortable to fly in first or business class than in economy class or on a charter flight. But most of us are willing to put up with a few hours of discomfort to get to our destination quickly and cheaply.

However you fly, sitting inactively for hours on end is risky – and the risk is not just of ankles and feet so swollen you can't get your shoes back on. Deep Vein Thrombosis – DVT, now commonly known as 'economy class syndrome' – is not confined to the back of the plane. Even those flying in comparative luxury are at risk. But everyone can reduce their chance of suffering from DVT by moving about the plane whenever possible and by doing a few simple exercises. For those passengers who are cramped and cannot leave their seats without disturbing other passengers, these exercises could even save lives.

DVT – what it means

A DVT is a blood clot that forms in a vein, most commonly in the deep vein of the calf. It causes pain and swelling, but more seriously, the clot can break away and lodge in the lungs as a potentially fatal pulmonary embolism. Blood is pumped from the heart round the body in arteries and is helped on its way by the muscular arterial wall. Veins return de-oxygenated blood to the right side of the heart which then pumps it to the lungs where it is loaded up with more oxygen.

Veins do not have a muscular wall to pump the blood back to the heart. The deep veins in the leg have valves and normally require assistance from the calf and other lower leg muscles to pump the blood onwards. Without this help, the blood within those veins slows down and a clot may form. This is why inactivity – being in bed after an operation, for example, or having to sit still for long periods – is conducive to the formation of DVT.

In hospitals, the incidence of DVT has been reduced by getting patients to wear special elasticated stockings which provide pressure to help keep the blood flowing in the veins. Wearing such stockings in planes would help to reduce swelling in travellers' legs, but they are expensive and difficult to put on. Women can wear support tights – the firmer the better – as a substitute for proper anti-embolism stockings. This is recommended for those who are at particular risk from DVT. Support tights are indistinguishable from normal tights in appearance and so look perfectly normal for women; they aren't normally worn by men, but (apart from the difficulty of finding tights big enough to fit most men) there's no good reason why they should not be put on under trousers.

There are a number of predisposing conditions which increase the risk of DVT:

POSSIBLE PRE-EXISTING INDIVIDUAL RISK FACTORS

→ Having had a DVT before
→ Having a rare genetic condition where the blood clots too readily
→ Being aged over 40
→ Being pregnant or taking hormone therapy (eg contraceptive pill or HRT)
→ Having had recent injury or surgery to the lower legs

→ Having varicose veins, heart failure or cancer
→ Being dehydrated (because of diarrhoea, for example)

FACTORS RELATING TO THE FLIGHT

→ The length and frequency of journeys
→ Reduced oxygen level
→ A cramped position – especially if asleep with the feet down
→ Being dehydrated (because of excessive alcohol)
→ Direct pressure on the veins in the calves from crossing legs or from the seats
→ Sitting still

Symptoms of DVT include swollen ankles and feet, and possibly some calf pain (although it should be stressed that some swelling of the ankles and feet need not mean that you have suffered a DVT).

The real danger from DVT is that part of the clot can be dislodged and be carried up to and through the heart and from there into the lungs – what is known as a pulmonary embolism. Symptoms include shortness of breath, grey pallor and sweating, and chest pain. This condition is potentially fatal – but thankfully it is also extremely rare. It can also be treated – as DVT can be treated – by anticoagulant therapy. But as this involves going to hospital, it is important to do everything in your power to prevent DVT in the first place.

Most airlines do their best to make flights safe and enjoyable for all their passengers. After all, happy passengers are more likely to travel with them again in the future. However, passengers also have a responsibility to behave in a way that is not only in their own best interest, but also does not interfere with other passengers or the flight and cabin crew.

The main purpose of this little book is to help you to prevent DVT and other, less serious, circulatory problems. But I hope the other information I have included will help make your whole trip more enjoyable so that when you reach your destination you are in your prime, and not dehydrated and weak like a wilted flower.

Travel preparations

Even before you set off for your flight, there are various matters that may affect how you feel during and after your journey. Feeling good is not just physical; there is a mental aspect to it, too, and every aspect of what makes you who you are must work together in a holistic way to ensure your well-being. Your hope, and the aim of this book, is that you will arrive at your destination in top form, physically and mentally. Minor irritations – from delays to having difficulty in finding your luggage on arrival – can raise your blood pressure and alter the way you feel.

Luggage

Heaving awkward, heavy luggage can cause back strain; even if you use a trolley, there is still some muscle work involved. Remember – this starts at home as you begin to get your cases ready for your journey.

TIPS ON LIFTING SAFELY

→ Plan the movement in advance – go the easiest route.

→ Breathe out, then pull your tummy in. Try to keep it pulled in throughout. The abdominal muscles are nature's corset and help to prevent damage to the spine.

→ Have your feet wide apart, keep your back straight and bend your knees so that they go directly over your feet.

➤ Reverse the sequence above when you
   lower the luggage.

TIPS ON LUGGAGE

➤ If you can cope with minimalist travel
   needs, and want to avoid waits in the
   baggage hall, take hand luggage only.
   Check with the airline exactly what size of
   case is allowed on-board.
➤ Keep the weight of the case, and its
   contents, to a minimum.
➤ Use a collapsible trolley or a case with
   wheels.
➤ For your return flight, make sure your case
   is big enough to cope with purchases made
   while away; or pack a smaller suitcase
   inside a larger one if you plan on a
   spending spree.

→ Make sure your case is sturdy and that zips, hinges and locks are in good condition. Use a strong luggage strap on the outside to prevent accidental opening and to help you identify your case easily. You can also use coloured tape or patches to aid identification on the carousel.

→ Keep heavy stuff like shoes at the bottom and back end of your case. Fill the corners.

→ Label your case clearly – but, for security reasons, do not have your home address on the outside of the case.

What to wear when you're six miles high

It's important to be comfortable on your flight – tight clothing is therefore not a good idea on a long flight. Remember, comfort is more important than appearance. But your chances of being upgraded might diminish if you turn up in a tracksuit. (I try to look smart for check-in but remove the formal layer once on the plane. If you already have a first-class ticket, it doesn't matter what you wear!) Remember, if you are at particular risk of DVT (see pages 11–12), it's a good idea to wear support tights.

Hand baggage

→ Select a bag that is easy to carry. A backpack is kinder to your spine than an ordinary bag as it keeps you balanced and disperses the weight in the most efficient way. Remember you might need extra space for things you buy in the airport shops.

→ If your destination has a very different climate from your place of departure, keep with you appropriate clothing for your arrival. This could mean stripping off an outer layer (and having enough room in your bag to store it) or having warm clothing in your bag for use on arrival.

→ If you are taking medication, keep two or three days' worth in your hand baggage in case the rest of your luggage gets lost or there are delays that result in an overnight stop when you can't get into your main baggage. (For the same reason, it's a good idea to keep a change of underwear, a T-shirt and a toothbrush in your hand baggage.)

→ For flights lasting over two hours, make sure you have enough reading or listening material with you for the journey (and for any delays). Remember, not all airlines or routes have in-flight videos; or you may already have seen the film. (In any case, if I watch the in-flight screen for too long, I get bad-tempered and prone to a headache.)

➤ If you want to sleep during the flight, take an inflatable pillow, eyeshades and earplugs (or headphones) with you in case these are not provided for your use.

➤ If you take your shoes off during a long flight, an extra pair of thick socks will make it easier to walk around the plane.

Travelling with children

If you are travelling with children, do not rely on the airline providing anything (although crew are generally very good with children). Some airlines supply meals only to passengers who have paid a proper fare, and children under two who travel for a fraction of a full fare may not get fed.

It is perfectly normal for young children to cry at take-off and landing – due to pressurisation changes – but you would hope they would not cry at other times. Parents need to plan ways to keep their children quietly occupied. Take pens, paper, games, books and puzzles in your hand-baggage (but not with lots of little pieces that could get lost).

Older children should be able to travel with decorum. Sometimes other passengers can be unsympathetic to parents and children – they don't understand how exhausting it can be to travel with young children and how difficult it can be to keep fractious children occupied for hours at a time. Most parents will be embarrassed (and in despair) if they cannot keep their children quiet, but if a child cries it could be because of illness, tiredness or fear. In these cases, it is not acceptable for other passengers to complain about the child's crying; it can even be counter-productive.

If your child needs a buggy, you may be allowed to take it to the departure gate. This makes it much easier to walk around the airport before you leave. But check with the airline where you can take your buggy. If you plan to use a taxi or a car on your arrival, you should take a car seat for safety with you (unless you know you can hire one at your destination – check this in advance). The car seat can be checked in with the rest of your baggage but it might need to be in protective wrapping.

From home to cabin seat

Plan it in advance. Visualise it

Plan how and when you are going to get to the airport at least the day before you travel. (Some people, like me, hate to hang around the airport a moment longer than necessary; others, like my husband, prefer to get there early enough to avoid any rush, before the check-in queue builds up, and to allow plenty of travel time in case of traffic jams and so on. I have to admit, the only times we have been upgraded are when he has won the argument about when to leave for the airport.)

Your check-in time can vary from 1 to 3 hours before departure. Your ticket or itinerary will tell you what it is and what the latest permissible time is.

Think about how you are going to get to the airport. Public transport can be unreliable. Taxis occasionally do not turn up. If you decide to drive yourself, allow plenty of time for this and for parking when you get to the airport, as this can take longer than you imagine. (If you opt for the cheaper parking remember that it will be further away from the departures terminal and you will have to rely on a shuttle bus to get you there. If you are travelling with your family, should you drop them off first with all your luggage at the terminal so that they can join the check-in queue while you park? Or should you all stay together all the way?)

Will you need a trolley? Who is going to find one? There are usually plenty of free trolleys at car parks, stations and other drop-off points. Who is going to carry what? (And do remember to use safe lifting techniques when you are moving your luggage on and off the trolley.)

The answer to all these questions is **visualisation**. If you are a seasoned traveller you will already know where to go and what works best. Otherwise, you will need to plan it all beforehand – time it all out, starting at check-in time and working backwards. If you have never been to this particular airport, make enquires (you can phone the airline or speak to seasoned travellers) before you plan your departure time.

LAST-MINUTE CHECKS
BEFORE YOU LEAVE HOME

➤ Have you cancelled deliveries (milk, newspapers etc)?

➤ If you have pets, have you made arrangements for them to be looked after?

➤ Have you left details of your itinerary and contact details with family and/or friends?

➤ Have you organised travel insurance (including adequate medical cover) – and have you packed copies of the documentation?

➤ Have you organised currency/traveller's cheques and remembered to take it/them?

➤ Have you kept your tickets and passports (and visas if required) in a convenient, secure but accessible place?

Checking in

When you arrive in the departures building, look for the monitors or screens that indicate where you will find your check-in desk. In large airports, this will be indicated on the right hand side of the screen. There may be several flights to the destination you are flying to – so make sure you have the correct airline, flight number and departure time.
(Sometimes only one or two desks are allocated to a particular flight; sometimes up to 20 desks will cope with flights by the same airline to many destinations. Sometimes there is a separate queue for each desk and sometimes there is one long zig-zag queue for a number of desks.)

At some airports, especially abroad, you are expected to get security clearance for your luggage (usually by putting it through an X-ray machine) before you go to the check-in desk.

Seating on board

Nowadays, seats are often allocated when you book your ticket. It is still sometimes possible to change your seat when you check in (but not if you turn up at the last minute).

Sitting in a window seat will mean that you will have to disturb at least one other passenger if you need to get up from your seat for any reason. On the other hand, you may prefer to sit by the window where nobody else needs to wake you or disturb you if they need to leave their seat. If you do not plan on moving during the flight, you *must* do Exercise 1 (see pages 46–49) to help prevent DVT.

An aisle seat will allow you to move about the plane more easily and sometimes stretch your legs a bit further.

Once you have checked in, you may have to wait for some time before it is time to board – time to shop if you want to. Airports often have two shopping areas – one before you go through security, the other after you have been through passport control (supposedly duty-free and often quite extensive but expensive). Do not get too carried away by duty-free. Is it worth the hassle to carry all those breakable, heavy goods in your hand baggage? And make sure the discounts are real!

In some countries, such as the United States, airlines have their own terminals which are sometimes quite small with no shopping or refreshment facilities. If you are in any doubt, ask about what is available before you go through security.

Hanging around

Check the monitor screens to see if your flight is functioning normally or whether it has been delayed. If a departure gate is listed, make sure you know how to get there (and how long it will take). Ask at the information desk if you're in doubt. Some gates are a long way away, so use a trolley if you can for heavy hand luggage.

It is imperative that you get to the gate early enough. Passengers must be at the gate at least 20 minutes before the listed departure time.

International law stipulates that a plane can take off only if all passengers who have checked baggage in are on board. Failure to turn up at the gate on time will result in the baggage being removed from the plane, and the flight being delayed; this may cause the flight to miss its departure slot and may incur considerable extra cost for the airline. This does not help to keep fares low. Plan your hanging-around time – and do not forget to go to the gate on time.

If you are going to be flying for more than five hours, have something light to eat and drink before you embark. You are unlikely to get a meal for at least an hour after take-off on a long-haul flight.

Listen to announcements, even if they are sometimes difficult to understand. You might have mislaid something vital (your boarding card, for example) and you could be being paged.

Walk around the lounges (or walk to your departure gate, especially if it is at some distance from the lounge) – this exercise will stimulate your circulation before your flight.

Large planes are usually loaded in sections, by row number. Your seat is reserved; so don't over-exert yourself to get on early. But remember that if you are too casual about this, other passengers may have filled the overhead lockers with their hand luggage before you get to your seat. If this is the case, the flight attendants will help find you storage space nearby.

In the air

Finally you are on the plane and in your seat. Loosen any tight clothing, especially socks. Avoid having anything that could impede circulation pressing into your lower legs.

Try to avoid having to open the overhead bins during the flight. Something could fall out. This could be embarrassing, but more seriously, it could be dangerous if something heavy fell on one of your fellow passengers. So before stowing your hand baggage, remember to take out anything you will need for the journey –

you can keep it in a small bag, under the seat in front of you or in your seat pocket.

WHAT YOU MIGHT NEED
DURING THE FLIGHT

→ Medicines – both prescription and 'comfort' ones
→ A pen to fill in landing documentation, visa forms (you will also need your passport, or notes of the relevant details, for this)
→ A personal stereo player and CDs or tapes
→ Tissues (temperature changes can make you sneeze)
→ Reading material and writing paper if you are likely to use it
→ Socks (if you are going to take your shoes off)
→ A mask, inflatable pillow and earplugs if you plan to sleep (check with the airline

whether these things are provided on your flight)

→ Credit card or money for on-board purchases

→ Clothing to help you warm up or cool down on the flight

→ A bottle of water on a long-haul flight (remember to drink lots of non-alcoholic drinks!)

→ Any work you may want to do during the flight. Check with the flight attendants whether and when laptops, mobile phones and other electronic equipment can be used.

→ If you are travelling with children, you will need things to keep them entertained and perhaps food, too, to keep them happy. Take lots of wet wipes, or a damp face-flannel. The flight attendants may help you to store such items as your baby's bottles of milk.

→ Remember in economy class that there is limited space.

Comfort on board

Pay attention to the safety demonstration just before take-off and read the safety card in the seat pocket in front of you. Once the plane has taken off, you can settle down comfortably and remove your shoes if you wish (but be sure to put them back on before landing).

Long-haul airlines usually provide pillows and blankets (one per person in economy, as many as you want in superior class). Sometimes your elbows can get somewhat tender because of the weight of your arm on the hard surface of the armrest – you can prevent this by putting a pillow under your elbow. (Of course, if you know the person you are sitting beside well

DO NOT CROSS YOUR LEGS – this compresses the blood vessels at the back of your legs and predisposes to swollen feet and ankles and the development of clots. You can cross your ankles. Do make sure that your socks are not constrictive at the top as this could impede your circulation. Shortly after take-off, when the cabin crew start to move around, you might want to remove your shoes.

enough, you can always lift the armrest between you.)

If you have a bad back, you might find it helpful to put a pillow behind the small of your back for extra support.

Remember to do Exercise 1 (*Tip Tap Rock* – see page 46) every 30–40 minutes when awake.

Seat belts

Most airlines ask you to keep your seat belt fastened all the time you are in your seat. This is a precaution against the unlikely case of sudden air turbulence which can be scary when it happens but is only really dangerous in severe cases when you are not strapped in. (In this case the turbulence could force you up and out of your seat and – very rarely indeed – cause you to bang your head on the ceiling.)

Make sure your seat belt is clearly visible to the flight crew if you want to sleep – fasten it on top of any blanket you are using – or you will be woken up if the seat belt sign is switched on. (And remember to let the flight crew know if you want to sleep during a meal service so that they do not wake you up.)

Service on board

Even the flight crew must remain seated until the plane has completed its initial steep climb. There will be no cabin service during this time – so do not ring the call bell unless there is a real emergency.

It is very easy to become dehydrated during flights – so drink as much water and soft drinks as you can. Excessive alcohol consumption adds to dehydration (ask anyone with a hangover – the headache and the dry feeling in the mouth!). It is very unwise to drink more than a little alcohol, even if it is free. Remember, dehydration is one of the factors that make it more likely for clots to form.

Remember, too, that excessive alcohol consumption could lead to aggressive and abusive behaviour towards other passengers or cabin crew. There is never any excuse for this, and in the confined space of a plane, it could also be dangerous, could lead to the plane being diverted to make an unscheduled landing for the unruly passengers to be expelled. This leads to more delay for everyone else and greater costs for the airline – for which the deportee could be liable. Do not risk getting a criminal record by drinking too much!

Food on board

On flights longer than four hours, most airlines will serve two meals, as well as drinks in between. This is usually one substantial meal and a snack just before landing. If you have any special dietary requirements, you should order a meal when booking your ticket – or up to 48 hours before the flight.

Fighting boredom – in-flight entertainment

Most airlines offer both audio and video entertainment (and sometimes computer games, too) for all passengers. Headphones which plug into the control panel on your seat arm are provided.

If you prefer to read, you can do so even when the main cabin lights are turned off, thanks to individual reading lights. These don't overly disturb other passengers who are trying to sleep (although the passenger who wants to sleep may still find a mask helpful).

Vary your activities. Too much reading or too much screen-watching can cause a headache. Don't forget the audio entertainment – this is (obviously) more restful for your eyes.
Also, provided the aisles are empty, it is a good idea occasionally to take a short walk. It provides some exercise and breaks the monotony of sitting.

Long flights are not a great pleasure to me or to many other people. But I hope the tips in this chapter and the exercises which follow will help to make it all less tiresome

The exercises

There are different reasons for doing each of the following exercises, but they all relate to keeping you comfortable and fit while in the air and having you in top form when you land. The most important of them is the first exercise, *TipTap Rock* – its purpose is to improve lower limb circulation and minimise the risk of DVT. This exercise is strongly recommended for everybody, and should be repeated every 30–40 minutes when you are awake. The others, whether done sitting down or standing in the aisle, are a menu from which you can select according to their different purposes.

It is better to do the exercises to appropriate music, either from the in-house audio tracks or from a personal tape or CD player. An indication of an optimum rhythm is given for each exercise.

None of these exercises should cause any pain.
They should be done gently and smoothly and should feel reasonably comfortable and natural. If there is any pain – stop. You may sometimes feel your muscles working (especially in *Tip Tap Rock*) but that is a different sensation from pain.

Exercises to do in your seat

EXERCISE 1: TIP TAP ROCK

Reasons for doing it: to improve circulation, prevent swollen ankles and DVT.

Starting position: sit up straight in your seat with your heels underneath your knees. Put your hands on your thighs.

Suggested rhythm: salsa beat.

> **Note:** When you are awake, repeat this exercise every 30–40 minutes. Do it when you first wake up.

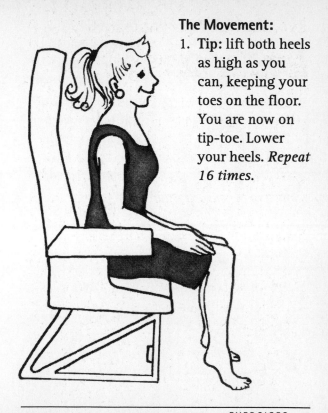

The Movement:

1. **Tip:** lift both heels as high as you can, keeping your toes on the floor. You are now on tip-toe. Lower your heels. *Repeat 16 times.*

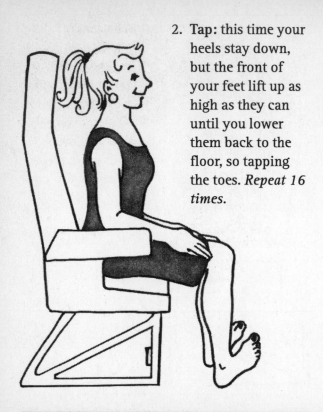

2. **Tap:** this time your heels stay down, but the front of your feet lift up as high as they can until you lower them back to the floor, so tapping the toes. *Repeat 16 times.*

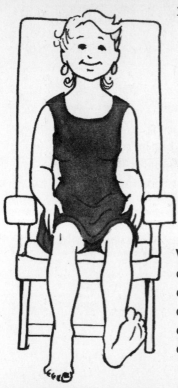

3. **Rock:** alternate the first two movements so that you lift your heels then tap your toes. In other words, you are rocking through your feet. *Repeat 16 complete movements.*

Variation: your feet can move in unison, or in opposing directions (so that one goes up as the other goes down).

EXERCISE 2: SHOULDER SHRUGS

Reasons for doing it: to reduce tension in the neck and shoulders.

Starting position: sit up as straight as possible, with your head against the seat (you may need a pillow). Think tall, but be relaxed with your chin tucked in. Your head should not move at all, and remain in this position of good posture all the time.

Suggested rhythm: a slow version of 'My Darling Clementine'.

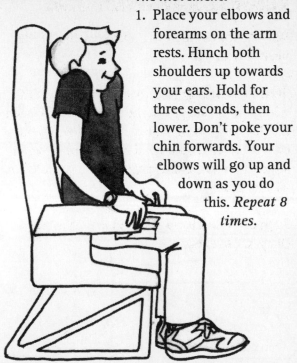

The Movement:

1. Place your elbows and forearms on the arm rests. Hunch both shoulders up towards your ears. Hold for three seconds, then lower. Don't poke your chin forwards. Your elbows will go up and down as you do this. *Repeat 8 times.*

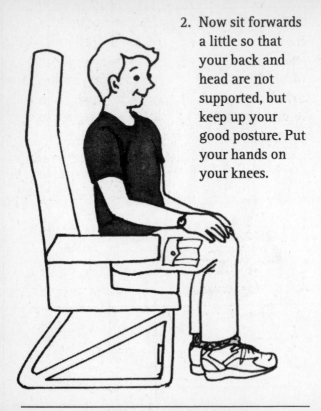

2. Now sit forwards a little so that your back and head are not supported, but keep up your good posture. Put your hands on your knees.

Slowly bring the front of your shoulders forwards so as to round them; return, then pull them backwards

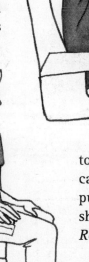

to brace, till you can feel a gentle pull between your shoulder blades. *Repeat 8 times.*

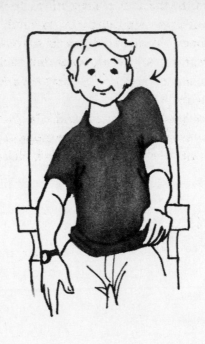

3. Combine the above two sections, to roll *one* shoulder in a slow circle by combining an up, back, down, and forwards movement. *Repeat 4 times, then change direction. Repeat the whole routine with the other shoulder.*
4. Move back in your seat, and relax, making sure that your shoulders are dropped down, your neck is long and your chin tucked in.

EXERCISE 3: THE CHARLESTON

Warning: if you have had bad arthritis in the hip, or have had a new hip joint within the past year, you should try this very gently and should not continue if there is any pain. **Do not do this exercise if you have an artificial knee joint.**

Reason for doing it: to mobilise the hip joints and work the abdominal muscles.

Starting position: Sit up straight with your thighs parallel, and your heels directly below your knees. This will mean your knees and feet (depending on how far apart your hips are) will be about 30 cm (12 ins) apart. Throughout the exercise, keep each knee at 90° (i.e., a right angle between calf and thigh).

Suggested rhythm: a slow Charleston.

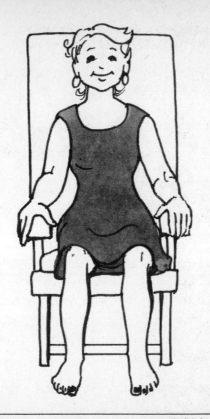

The Movement:

1. Pull in your tummy and lift both legs a little bit, put your feet down so that their undersides are touching each other and your knees are as far apart as possible.

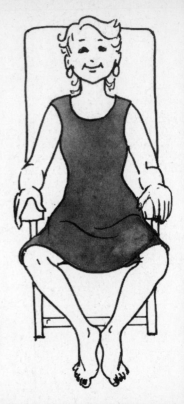

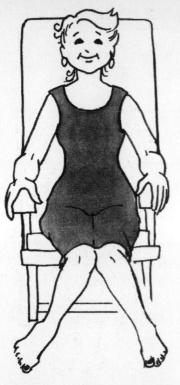

2. Still with your tummy in, lift your legs again, but this time reverse the movement, so that your knees (and thighs) are touching, but your feet are as far apart as possible.

3. Continue to 'Charleston' about 16 complete movements.

EXERCISE 4: PELVIC ROCKING

Reasons for doing it: to mobilise the lumbar spine and work the abdominal muscles.

Starting position: Sit upright in your seat, but a little way forwards, so that your back is not supported.

Suggested rhythm: a slow strip tease beat.

The Movement:
1. Breathe in. As you breathe out, pull in your tummy, as though trying to suck your belly button towards your spine. Keeping the tummy sucked in, carry on breathing normally. Do not hold your breath.

2. Still holding your tummy in, smoothly and gently, tuck in your bottom, to curve your lumbar spine backwards – till you can feel your back touch the seat.

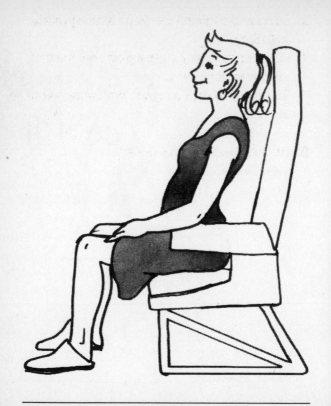

3. Reverse the movement so as to sit upright, as before.
4. Carry on to gently so that you now have a hollow in your back.
5. Repeat slowly curving and hollowing about 8 times.

Remember – nothing should hurt.

EXERCISE 5:
HAND AND FOOT SQUEEZES

Reasons for doing it: to work the arm and leg muscles (biceps, triceps, quadriceps and hamstrings); to build up tension, and then to release it and get the relaxation afterwards.

Starting position: Sit up straight, with your back supported. Make your hands into fists, and put the right fist on top of the left one, so that the thumbs are uppermost. Hold your arms at waist level.

Suggested rhythm: instead of music, think of counting 5–10 seconds for each hold.

The Movement:

1. Press the two fists together as hard as you can – but without moving your elbows. This is a static muscle contraction. Keep the pressure up for 5–10 seconds, but don't hold your breath. *Repeat 5 times, then change over your hands so that the left is on top.*

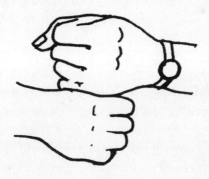

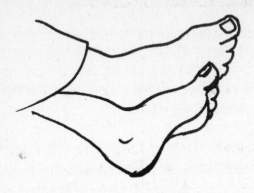

2. Cross your feet just above the ankles, and then lift them as high as space permits. Press the two ankles together as hard as you can – without moving your knees. Keep the pressure up for 5–10 seconds, but again, don't hold your breath. *Repeat 5 times.*

3. Try to do both fist and ankle squeezes at the same time. *Repeat 5 times.*

EXERCISE 6: NECK BENDS

Reasons for doing it: To increase neck mobility and reduce tension.

Starting position: Sit back in your seat, with your shoulders relaxed.

Suggested rhythm: Imagine singing up a scale of one octave, and then down again. Each individual movement should last that long.

continued overleaf

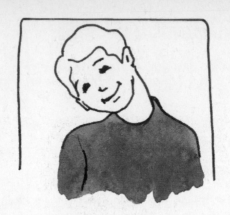

The Movement:

1. **Tip:** Keeping your shoulders facing forward and relaxed, slowly tip your head to one side, as though you are trying to get your ear to touch your shoulder. Your head should not turn, but only tip (like a budgie!). *Repeat 4 times then change sides.*

2. **Turn:** This time you turn your head to one side, as far as you can. You can even give

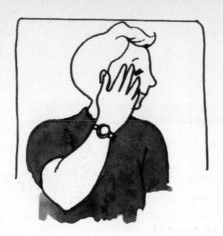

gentle overpressure with your hand. *Repeat as above.*

3. **Stretch:** Lastly, try to make your neck a little longer, by sliding the back of your head a couple of millimetres up the back of the seat, whilst gently pulling your chin in as though to make a double chin. *Repeat slowly five times.*

> **Note:** The next two exercises require space above your head and it may therefore not be possible to do them in some seats.

EXERCISE 7: BODY BOWING

Reasons for doing it: To stretch and move the arm and spine.

Starting position: Sit up straight in your seat with both arms straight, above your head, with palms touching.

Suggested rhythm: very slow.

The Movement:
Stretch your right hand even higher above your head, as though trying to reach for the sky. In order to get a bit further, when stretching your right arm up, shift your weight

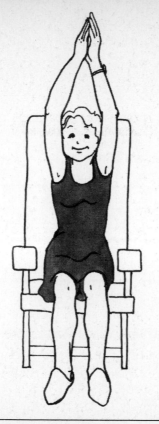

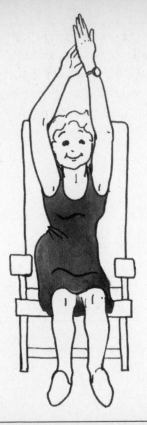

onto the right hip, and off the left hip. You should be able to get your right hand higher than your left. You will find that your spine is curving sideways. Now repeat the process, but with your left hand stretching. *Repeat 4 times to each side.*

EXERCISE 8: ARM AND HAND STRETCH

Reasons for doing it: To mobilise and stretch the shoulders and arms.

Starting position: Again, sit up straight in your seat. Interlock your fingers above your head, so that the backs of your hands are facing upwards.

The Movement:
Keeping your fingers interlocked, lower your hands a little, then turn both palms forwards and upwards, until your palms are facing up. If you can, keep your elbows straight and stretch your arms as far back as possible. You will feel a stretch in both arms, but do not push into pain. Hold the stretch for about 5–10 seconds. *Repeat once or twice.*

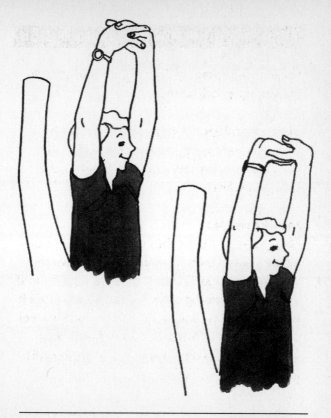

EXERCISE 9: RELAXATION AND DEEP BREATHING

Reasons for doing it: To reduce tension, to increase oxygen levels in the blood, and to promote relaxation. This exercise is useful for nervous moments, like take-off, landing or during turbulence. By concentrating inwardly on promoting pleasant physical sensations, you can shut out negative thoughts and anxieties.

Starting position: Sit supported in your seat, as comfortable as possible. Perhaps with pillows behind your head, and/or under your elbows. Close your eyes.

Suggested music: something very slow and sleepy, which you really like. Some airlines'

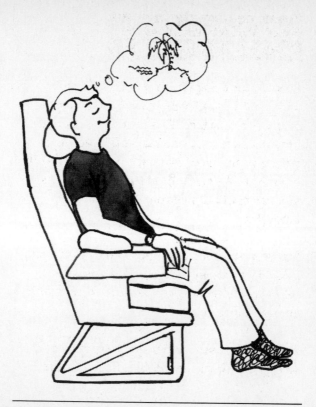

audio systems have a channel dedicated to relaxing music. (My personal choice is the slow movement of any of Mozart's piano concertos, especially the 19th.)

The Movement:
1. This time there is no movement. The idea is to relax, to reduce all muscle tension. Think about breathing slowly, concentrating more on breathing out than in. Count slowly as you inhale for 2 and then exhale for 5.
2. Imagine you are in your favourite, happiest, most relaxing place. Perhaps it is a holiday, a tropical beach, the countryside – anywhere you can visualise. In your mind's eye, imagine a place where you have been, perhaps with someone you love. Listen to the bird-songs, the sound of the sea or the noise of children playing – whatever is relevant to your special place and time.

Synchronise nature's rhythms with your slowed-down breathing. Concentrate on what the smell would be – but always think of happy, enjoyable sensations.

3. Some people find it helps to relax muscles after first building up the tension. Just once, clench your fists, arms and legs really tight (as in Exercise 5), but hold it all for only two or three seconds. Then let go and feel the release. Try letting go a bit further so that anybody prodding you would feel a softness (as compared to the tension when you did Exercise 5). Carry on this feeling of releasing even further, until you feel that you are floating on a cloud. When you are really relaxed, you feel weightless, but you also feel as though you are deeply asleep, and very heavy. It is almost as though you have too much inertia to move. You are outside your body watching it float away.

When relaxed, there is a sensation of allowing somebody else to move your limbs, without your helping or hindering them.

Note: Being able to relax mentally and physically at will is a very valuable and health-promoting resource. It can help to reduce blood pressure, reduce tension at work and minimise pain.

Exercises to do when standing in the aisles

> **Warning:** Only do these exercises when the seat belt sign is off and only if you will not interfere with any trolley service that is in progress.

EXERCISE 10: THE CHANGES

Reasons for doing it: to provide a strong circulation pump for the legs to minimise swelling of the legs and so help prevent DVT.

Starting position: Stand with your feet about 30 cm (12 ins) apart, and hold onto the back of a seat, or put both hands on the wall at shoulder height. This exercise can usefully be done when you are queuing for the toilet.

Suggested rhythm:
A quick march
tempo.

The Movement:
1. Go up and down
   onto tip-toes,
   without bending
   your knees.
   Repeat 10 times.

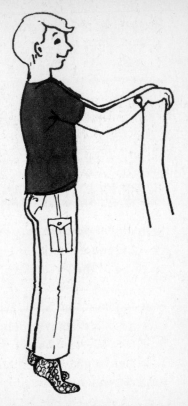

2. Now do the same movement, but make your calves work a bit harder by transferring your weight from one foot to the other. One foot remains flat while the other heel lifts up, making the knee go forward. Your head should also go up and down. All the time, your toes should be stuck to the floor. *Repeat 10 times with each foot.*

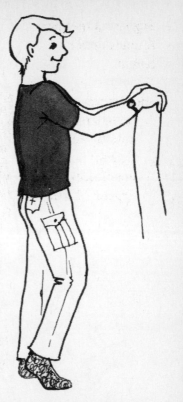

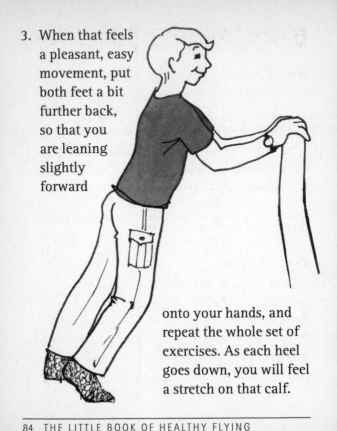

3. When that feels a pleasant, easy movement, put both feet a bit further back, so that you are leaning slightly forward

onto your hands, and repeat the whole set of exercises. As each heel goes down, you will feel a stretch on that calf.

EXERCISE 11: STANDING TIP TAP ROCK

Reasons for doing it: To stimulate circulation to minimise swollen feet and prevent DVT.

Starting position: Stand with your feet a little way apart but hold on firmly to the back of a seat, or something solid (but not the handle of the emergency exit!)

Suggested rhythm: Salsa beat.

The Movement:
This is a repeat of Exercise 1, but done standing instead of sitting. See pages 46–49 for detailed instructions. The tip-toe is easy, but it is hard not to fall backwards when you 'tap' – that is why you need to hold on. When combining the movements into a full rock, it is

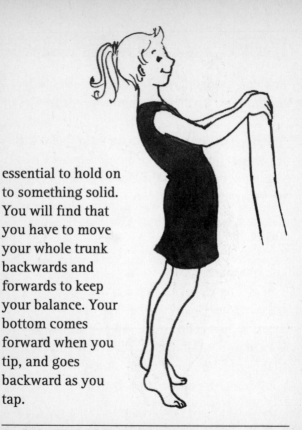

essential to hold on to something solid. You will find that you have to move your whole trunk backwards and forwards to keep your balance. Your bottom comes forward when you tip, and goes backward as you tap.

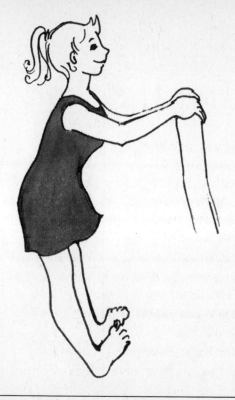

After the flight

Getting off the plane

When the Captain announces that the plane will shortly be landing, it is time to put on your shoes. If you have continued to do the Tip Tap Rock exercise, the swelling in your feet and ankles should be minimal. You are usually given about 30 minutes notice of landing, and this should be ample time to get your shoes on and get your papers organised.

You will also have time for a clothing adjustment – to remove a layer of clothing or your tights before you land somewhere very hot, for example. If you don't manage to do this on the plane, you can always do it in the arrival terminal when you get there.

Pay attention to any pre-landing video the airline shows – it may contain useful information about the arrival procedures at your destination airport

Remember to have your passport accessible, together with any visas, immigration or customs papers you will need. Also keep a pen handy in case of last-minute form-filling.

Passengers are disembarked according to class of travel. So if you are travelling at the rear of the economy section in a jumbo, it will take about 15 minutes for you to get off after the plane becomes stationary.

Do you really need to stand up and get your possessions out of the overhead lockers as soon as the seat belt sign is turned off? If you are by a window, you may not even be able to stand fully erect.

Even though the actual disembarkation process is usually remarkably orderly, and people do seem to allow those who are seated in front of them to get off first, the aisles are narrow and people are often encumbered with awkward hand baggage, so you can expect to be caught up in a fast-flowing river of single-minded people. Therefore, if you are travelling with children or are at all unsteady or fragile, it is much wiser to sit down and wait for the other passengers to leave first. This will take only a few extra minutes.

Getting to immigration and baggage collection in the terminal

In many airports you will have quite a long walk to get to Immigration. Walking is very good for your circulation, so even if there are travelators, it is advisable to walk at least some of the way – or to walk while on the travelator.

Try to get to Immigration as quickly as you can – to minimise the amount of time you will have to wait. This varies greatly from country to country, and can also depend on the size of plane and whether more than one flight has landed around the same time.

Even if you are exhausted, try to be courteous and good-humoured with the officials: this will help you to remain calm, will help to keep your blood pressure down, and might even speed things up.

Baggage

Look out for the monitors indicating which carousel your flight's baggage will be delivered to. Luggage trolleys are usually available, although sometimes you have to pay for these in local currency. (Seasoned travellers always keep a cache of foreign small change at home – in some places, the exchange office may be

---

Remember to keep your back straight and bend your knees when lifting cases from the carousel to the trolley. Also, ensure that the trolley is not going to move as you are putting your case on. Either get someone else to hold it still, or wedge it against the side of the carousel.

---

closed, or it may only be possible to buy currency after you have left the baggage hall. You might also need some local currency if you are planning to take a taxi from the airport.)

To save a few moments watching your cases slowly revolve, take your trolley to the point nearest to where the luggage appears.

Return flights

Some airlines ask that your re-confirm your return flights 2 or 3 days before you are due to return. If you are in any doubt about this, check with an official of your airline while you are at the airport.

If you were not happy with the meals you were given during your flight, you might want to order a special meal for the return flight. Major

airlines offer a variety of special meals –
vegetarian, vegan, kosher, hallal, etc. – but
they all require at least 48 hours notice. It may
be possible – and easier – to do this at the
airport when you have cleared customs on
your arrival.

Transport from the airport

If you are on a package holiday, onward travel
to your hotel will probably have been
organised for you, and if you are lucky, this
will be by taxi, special car or minibus.
Sometimes, a series of coaches are arranged to
drop passengers off at their hotels. This can
mean hanging around in the coach for quite a
long time until it is fully loaded and sometimes
the luck of the draw will mean that your hotel
is the last on the list.

If you are making an overnight or one-day stop, you should consider taking your immediate requirements in your hand baggage and checking your main baggage into a left-luggage locker at the airport. Better still, when you check in at your first departure, find out if you can check your bags through to your final destination. This can often be arranged if your stop-over is less than 24 hours, and if your continuation is on the same airline. This offers huge savings of time and emotional effort.

Hassle factor

In many parts of the world, you can emerge from the Customs Hall to face a barrage of taxi drivers or 'entrepreneurial' middlemen touting for your business. You may have to haggle over the fare.

If you are not being met, go to the information desk before you go outside to find out what transport is available, what it should cost, and whether there are officially recognised vehicles.

Ask about local tipping customs. And make sure you have local currency readily available for your taxi driver or the porter at your hotel.

So – have a great trip, and may it achieve all your planned objectives.